THE MENTAL HEALTH OF EVANGELICAL PASTORS

Delcio Torres Amorim Junior

English Version

The mental health of evangelical pastors. English version. Delcio Torres Amorim Junior. Londrina-Brazil. Edições Universo Teológico. 2022.
100 pp:14x21 cm
ISBN:
All rights reserved to the author
Partial reproduction allowed if the source is identified

1. Mental Health 2. Pastor 3. Aflictions 4. Provisions from God

SUMARY

1. INTRODUCTION 08
2. HOW ARE PASTORS FEELING? 10
3. BUT, WHY PASTORS CAN SUFFER? 14
4. THE PROFESSION-MINISTRY BINOMIAL 16
5. WHICH ARE THE PASTOR'S AFFLICTIONS? 20
6. AFFLICTIONS OF THE PASTOR'S FAMILY 26
7. THE PASTOR'S MENTAL HEALTH 28
8. ANXIETY DISORDERS 30
9. ANXIETY DISORDERS IN THE BIBLE 34
10. DEPRESSIVE DISORDERS 38
11. DEPRESSIVE DISORDERS IN THE BIBLE 42
12. BURNOUT SYNDROME 50
13. BURNOUT SYNDROME IN THE BIBLE 58
14. SUICIDE 60
15. PROVISIONS FROM GOD 62
16. THE DIVINE RESTORATION 66
17. LIFESTYLE CHANGES 70
18. PERSONAL SUPPORT 74
19. PROFESSIONAL SUPPORT 76
20. DRUG THERAPY 80
21. FINAL CONSIDERATIONS 84
ABOUT THE AUTHOR 86
REFERENCES 88

1. INTRODUCTION

Pastoral ministry requires a lot of activities and dedication from pastors and religious ministers to meet the needs, demands and expectations of the religious denomination, the church and its members, as well as regarding the local society. In addition to these, there are the pastor's own family that requires attention to the spouse and children, and the church's own demands and expectations in relation to the pastor's family demanding patterns of behavior and engagement in the church's activities as if pastors also were. These demands are so intense that they place a very heavy burden on the pastor's shoulders, producing physical, emotional and spiritual stress, increasing the risk of physical and mental illnesses. The reflection of this situation has appeared due to the increase in the number of pastors who leave the ministry, the incidence of mental disorders above those found in the general population and cases of suicide. Physical diseases (such as hypertension, dermatological disorders, obesity, diabetes mellitus, coronary heart disease and acute myocardial infarction, among others), have their causes mainly attributed to organic, physical and lifestyle factors (sedentary lifestyle, unbalanced diet, etc.). On the other hand, mental disorders instigate heated discussions and diverse points of view, as a rule, loaded with prejudice, religious dogmas, erroneous understanding of the Bible and lack of medical, psychological and scientific knowledge. Mental disorders within the church have not yet been considered and treated with the importance and complexity they deserve and demand (in most cases they are considered as spiritual failures, lack of relationship and intimacy with God or the practice of sin). But, on the other hand, this issue has been attracted attention of the academic world, researchers and health professionals with multiplication of research, publication of articles in indexed and impact journals, monographs of specialization courses, master's dissertations, doctoral theses and even post-doctoral research in internationally recognized secular universities.

The purpose of this book is to present a brief medical, psychological and theological approach to depression, anxiety disorders, burnout and suicide that affect reformed Christian pastors ("evangelical pastors"), as a way to demystify and break down paradigms about mental disorders, instigate and encourage discussions and reflections about the subject in churches.

2. HOW ARE PASTORS FEELING?

In 2016, Francis A. Schaeffer Institute of Church Leadership Development (www.churchleadership.org), published "Statistics on Pastors: 2016 Update – Research on the Happenings in Pastors' Personal and Church Lives". They conducted several major studies involving 8,150 participants, including those identified as Evangelical or Reformed. Data sources included long-form handouts, personal interviews, several social media polls and alternate email to check validity as well as to retest results from different samplings.
A brief overview of the statistics reveals that:

- 89% of pastors have already thought about leaving the ministry
- 57% would leave if they had a better place, including secular work
- 72% studied the Bible only when preparing studies or sermons
- 54% of pastors work over 55 hours a week
- 57% can not pay their bills
- 54% are overworked and 43% are overstressed
- 53% feel seminary had not properly prepared them for the task.
- 35% battle depression
- 26% are overly fatigued
- 28% are spiritually undernourished
- 9% are burned-out
- 23% are distant to their families

- 18% work more than 70 hours a week and face unreasonable challenges
- 12% are belittled
- 3% have had an affair

In addition, the researchers collected some insights from interview, consulting data, social media polls and pastors conference surveys, not indicative of a national random sampling like those above, but providing insights and warnings:

- Pastors are happier, but not healthier
- 65% of pastors feel their family is in a 'glass house' and fear they are not good enough to meet expectations.
- 65% of pastors do not feel their churches are in sync to their family needs.
- 44% of pastor's families are not pleased with their church.
- 24% of families resent the church and its effects on their family.
- 52% of pastors feel they are overworked and can not meet their church's unrealistic expectations.
- 66% of pastors feel their churches are not in sync to ministry agendas.
- 58% of pastors feel they do not have any good true friends.
- 58% of pastors feel their church does not empowers them to have a life outside of the church.

- 66% of pastors do not battle discouragement on a regular basis
- 35% of pastors battle depression or fear of inadequacy
- 27% of pastors stated they have no one to turn to if they are facing a crisis
- 40% of pastor's wives do not feel their church treats their family well
- 22% of pastor's wives feel the ministry places undue expectations on their family
- 26% of pastor's wives feel church is a prime source of stress for their family.
- 63% of pastor's wives feel finances is a prime source of stress for their family.
- An observation, not researched, of many pastors today, perhaps 50%, is that they are very unhealthy, overweight, with health problems stemming from poor food intake and excess junk food, a lack of exercise, and to a lesser extent, alcohol
- Three doctors who see a lot of pastors have told that there is a significant increase of hypertension, obesity, cardiovascular problems, and depression

This information is extremely worrying and gives an idea of the scale of the problem: unsound men and women, suffering emotional and spiritually, who have not been cared for, taking care of unsound people, who are emotional and spiritually suffering as well. It is the blind leading the blind! Disaster is inevitable. Everything is just a matter of time.

This scenario explains unhealthy churches, full of unhealthy members, guided by unhealthy leaders, who fail to enjoy the fullness of God's blessings, but only survive by God's mercy and grace.

3. BUT, WHY PASTORS CAN SUFFER?

Many people see religious leaders as "enlightened beings" who live in a higher dimension than other mortals do. They have the false vision and expectation that they are not the same as other people, with feelings, emotions, weaknesses and needs. In the view of these people, pastors (like other religious leaders) have the supernatural ability to detach themselves from emotions and worldly or material things, forgetting that they are just imperfect people who have chosen to serve a perfect God. Although they seek to be imitators of Christ, they are flawed and subject to emotions and will suffer all the afflictions common to anyone. Jesus knew this and warned his disciples.

"I have told you these things, so that in me you may have peace. In this world, you will have **TROUBLE**. But, take heart! I have overcome the world" (John 16.33 – New International Version - NIV)

In the Greek original version, "trouble" is the word "θλιψις" (*thlipsis*), which means the act of pressing, pressure (literally or figuratively). Metaphorically it can mean oppression, affliction, tribulation, burdened, persecution anguish and dilemmas. It is also synonymous with "στενοχωρια" (*stenochoria*) which means "narrow place". The prefix "θλι" (thli) composes the word "θλιβω" (*thlibo*), which means to press (like grapes in the winepress), to squeeze, to press firmly which, metaphorically means to bore, to afflict, anguish, narrow, throng, suffer tribulation, trouble.

In this way, "trouble" does not refer only to the difficult or unpleasant everyday situations of life, but to circumstances and situations that limit one's own life, as if one is being pressed like a grape in the winepress (Strong Dictionary). However, Jesus also made the promise that he is our source of provisions for us to go through these situations.

4. THE PROFESSION-MINISTRY BINOMIAL

When it comes to pastoral activity, as a rule, ministry is considered as selflessness and dedication to a cause or ideal (in this case, preaching the Gospel and helping the needy "*lato sensu*"), disregarding the professional aspects of the pastor or religious minister. The view that the pastor is just an individual dedicated to caring for and caring for "spiritual things", "the things of God", "what comes from above", disregards pastoral activity, also, as a profession, with all the implications of a professional activity, including legal aspects. The pastor (comprising in this term all those who develop ministerial activity full or part time) is seen as a separate person to serve the church, people and the community without restrictions, and must be available at all times, regardless of their needs. They consist on socializing and family care, rest, emotional support, physical and mental health care, and, mainly, financial. There is a widespread and ingrained concept that "if God takes care of his children, he will take care of all the needs of those who proclaim his Word". Indeed, God takes care of his children; however, this care is not only supernaturally "*strictu sensu*", like manna spilled from heaven, but by the provision of "means", which include the care of the church with its pastors both spiritually as materially.

Paul, writing to the Hebrews, shows this need for spiritual coverage to the pastors by the church:

"Have confidence in your leaders and submit to their authority, because they keep watch over you as those who must give an account. Do this so that their work will be a joy, not a burden, for that would be of no benefit to you. Pray for us. We are sure that we have a clear conscience and desire to live honorably in every way. I particularly urge you to pray so that I may be restored to you soon" (Hebrews 13.17-19 - NIV).

Paul still writes about material support for preachers of the Gospel:

"I know what it is to be in need, and I know what it is to have plenty. I have learned the secret of being content in any and every situation, whether well fed or hungry, whether living in plenty or in want. I can do all this through him who gives me strength. Yet it was good of you to share in my troubles. Moreover, as you Philippians know, in the early days of your acquaintance with the gospel, when I set out from Macedonia, not one church shared with me in the matter of giving and receiving, except you only; for even when I was in Thessalonica, you sent me aid more than once when I was in need. Not that I desire your gifts; what I desire is that more be credited to your account. I have received full payment and have more than enough. I am amply supplied, now that I have received from Epaphroditus the gifts you sent. They are a fragrant offering, an acceptable sacrifice, pleasing to God" (Philippians 4.12-18 - NIV).

Despite his spiritual activity, the pastor is a human being who lives in the physical, material world, with equally spiritual and physical needs, including family and social, who carries out a professional activity, legally recognized as such.

5. WHICH ARE THE PASTOR'S AFFLICTIONS?

The lack of understanding of the ministry-profession binomial, even by the pastor himself, always produces some degree of suffering. In general, church members see the pastor as someone who is full time exclusively dedicated to the needs and demands of the church, regardless of the pastor's own needs. This generates explicit and non-explicit charges. It is as if pastoral activity implies detachment from one's own life, introjecting into the pastor's subconscious this type of demand on oneself, and the unconditional responsibility to meet the expectations of members (personal assistance, quantitative growth of the church, social works, respect and recognition of the church in the community, among other activities), take care of your personal needs. It remains for the pastor to "worry about things that come from above", without being careful about "things that are down here". These situations and demands produce afflictions, inner conflicts, "self-charges", which lead to suffering that, together with the lack of spiritual and emotional support, generates stress. In turn, constant stress triggers anxiety episodes that can produce a generalized anxiety disorder, limiting personal and professional activities and favoring other physical and mental health problems. People who suffer from generalized anxiety disorder are five times more likely to develop depression.

Handling conflicts is part of pastoral activity, and perhaps the one that takes the longest. Pastor attends to the most varied kinds of conflicts, such as problems between family members (spouses, parents and children, brothers), between church members, workers, volunteers and church employees. Pastor assumes the exhausting function of managing people in an environment in which the "pastor-pastor" is not often separated from the "manager-pastor", fighting against the expectations of alleviating conflicts ("going over the head") when in fact, more energetic attitudes and words are needed. Many people who are in churches, born into a Christian family, as well as converts to the Gospel, carry an emotional burden, often with trauma and important behavioral disorders that can profoundly affect their personal, professional and self-relationships. These behavioral aspects are often the very factor for conversion to the Gospel, but taken to the church as well. When not treated properly, they can affect relations between members, and cause dissensions and problems that affect the church itself (divisions, loss of members, adultery, fraud, unpaid debts, fraud, etc.). There is a mistaken belief that with the conversion to the Gospel the transformation of the character occurs automatically, when, in fact, the touch of the Holy Spirit raises awareness of sin and presents the saving power of Jesus' sacrifice on the cross, due to the infinite love of Jesus. God. From then on, the spirit surrenders to Christ, but the traumas and wounds in the soul (*psiché*) must still need to be treated in a process known as "inner healing". This healing process can be long and requires advice, monitoring, reading and meditation on the Word of God, much prayer, besides time and dedication, generating physical and emotional distress for the pastor himself. An aggravating factor in this matter is the fact that the pastor has his limitations of time availability, training in counseling and his own untreated inner wounds, further increasing his afflictions and anxieties to meet expectations. The existence of active, participatory leadership is of great importance to lighten the burden on the pastor's back.

Another important aspect concerns the pastor's own condition as a "professional". If, on the one hand, the pastor can be seen as an employee of the church and, therefore, liable to resignation, on the other, there is still the perception, in many churches, that the pastor is selfless, devoid of material needs and that survive only and exclusively by grace. These churches do not have a human resources policy with adequate remuneration that allows minimum conditions for the support of the pastor and his family, retirement plan (official or supplementary), health care, vacation and other labor rights, contrary to the Bible itself:

"The elders who direct the affairs of the church well are worthy of double honor, especially those whose work is preaching and teaching. For Scripture says, "Do not muzzle an ox while it is treading out the grain," and "The worker deserves his wages" (1 Timothy 5.17-18 - NIV).

In addition, there are no financial education programs to skill pastors on personal resources management and, eventually, those entrusted by the church:

"Why spend money on what is not bread, and your labor on what does not satisfy? Listen, listen to me, and eat what is good, and you will delight in the richest of fare" (Isaiah 55.2 - NIV).

In summary, the main pastor's afflictions:

- Problems with difficult and wearable people
- Temperament problems of the followers that hinder the ministry
- Insubordination that causes problems
- Financial difficulties
- The loneliness of pastoral ministry (Cassemiro, 2019)
- Less material compensation (wages and benefits) compared to other professionals with equivalent training and responsibility
- Restriction of personal pleasure
- Restriction of normal expression of emotions
- Lack of privacy with his personal life highly exposed
- Relationship with superiors (church council, presbytery, assembly of members, denominational structure)
- Wear and tear by the constant need to help people in their difficulties
- Expectation of members to have authority over all matters
- Difficulties in establishing limits, causing physical and mental exhaustion in addition to emotional imbalance
- Ministerial activism leading to loss of focus and objectives

- Considering that he should be spared from life's problems and difficulties due to dedicating himself to spiritual activity (Lotufo, 2009)
- Personal expectations of church growth
- The demand or need for mass evangelism in a church-company view
- Financial difficulties due to low pay or the inability to handle personal finances
- Instability in maintaining employment
- Afflictions of spouse and children (Bovo, 2019)

6. THE AFFLICTIONS OF THE PASTOR'S FAMILY

In the family environment, attitudes and situations involving one of its members directly or indirectly affect everyone. Joyful events (marriage, pregnancy, birth of a child, completion of a course, a new job) and sad events (death, marital separation, drug addiction, job loss, bankruptcy), interpersonal problems within and outside the family circle, they can deeply affect people, causing different levels of suffering with different reactions from each family member. This occurs regardless of the individual's career or profession. However, the pastor's family is particularly affected not only by the situations that affect families in general, but precisely by the fact that it is "the pastor's family", suffering constant "patrolling" and charges that are completely unacceptable or unreasonable, like no other is. Pastor's wife is expected to have the same ministry as her husband's. She is demanded to play an active role in the church in the same dimensions as the pastor. Her role as a helper in ministerial life, providing support and emotional security, taking care of physical and material needs (the governance of the house), the attention and care of children and, eventually, contributing to financial support, providing support for the exercise of pastoral ministry is neither considered nor valued. She is a constant target of criticism, whether for the absence in some church activity, for a style of clothing, for the type of hairstyle or makeup, for the availability of time to attend to people, for the way she educates her children, in short, for each gesture, act or word and, even, by silence. The pastor's children are also required to behave in terms of behavior, interpersonal relationships, participation in church activities and ministries as if "a pastor's son, pastor were", disrespecting individuality, preferences, aptitudes, talents and vocation (Vargas, 2019). This would be tantamount to requiring the doctor's wife to be a doctor and that all of her children are also doctors.

Pastor's family suffers from the absence or the little time dedicated by the pastor to them, due to the intense activities of the church, lack of moments of leisure and family life, financial difficulties, the heavy burden of charges. This lack of time for family's relationship needs causes physical and emotional stress throughout family nucleus, often leading to adultery, divorce and disinterest in children in church activities and even in Christ.

Family afflictions directly affect the pastor, increase the stress of an already stressful activity, compromise the performance of functions, causing anxiety that increases the likelihood of depression and physical and mental exhaustion (burn-out syndrome).

7. THE PASTOR'S MENTAL HEALTH

Many are the pastor's afflictions, from individual issues, past feelings and traumas, issues related to the exercise of pastoral activity and family, which act as stressors or cause some degree of suffering. Stressful working conditions involving activism with a lack of defined working hours, over-mediation of conflicts (as a trigger for bitterness and memories of the past), the unbridled pursuit of mass evangelization as a way for quantitative growth in the number of members, collecting tithes and job maintenance, are predisposing factors to extreme anxiety. Combination of all these factors can trigger psycho-emotional disorders that can deeply compromise pastor's life. Scientific literature shows that there is, "lato sensu", a negative correlation between religiosity or spirituality and mental health problems (those individuals adhering to a religion, especially non-Pentecostal Protestants, present a reduced risk of disorders psychiatric disorders, markedly alcoholism and drug addiction). Despite this fact, pastors, together with doctors, are at increased risk of affective and anxious disorders (LOTUFO, 2009. p. 257; SOEIRO et al, 2008), with emphasis on generalized anxiety disorder, the depression and burnout.

8. ANXIETY DISORDERS

Anxiety disorders are a group of mental and behavioral disorders characterized by feelings of excessive anxiety and fear. They include generalized anxiety disorder (GAD), panic disorder, phobias, social anxiety disorder, obsessive-compulsive disorder (OCD) and post-traumatic stress disorder, with mild to severe symptoms that persist for a long time (WHO, 2017). Fear is the emotional response to a real or perceived danger, current or ongoing, while anxiety is the anticipation of a future danger or threat, which can normally present themselves to anyone, as transient, adaptive conditions without major consequences. Anxiety disorders are different from adaptive fear and anxiety, normal in any life situations, as they are excessive or prolong (usually more than six months) interfering with the individual's normal life, usually induced by stress. Panic attacks are a particular type of response to fear and can be seen in other mental disorders too (DSM V, 2014).

High psychological demand, low pay, emotional demands and insecurity are predisposing factors for anxiety disorders (Fernandes et al, 2018). These disorders are the sixth cause of absence from work in the world and the third in the Americas (WHO, 2015). They are the most frequent psychiatric disorders in all age groups, being almost twice as prevalent in women as in men and have the following incidences:

- World: 3.6%
- Pacific West Coast: 2.9%

- Americas: 5.8%
- Brazil: 9.3% (WHO – OMS, 2015)
- Pastors: 11.1% (Duke Clergy Health Initiative, 2014).

Individuals suffering from generalized anxiety disorder (GAD) are at increased risk for other psychiatric disorders:

- Major depressive disorder: 53.7% of patients with GAD
- Suicide: 54.8% of patients with GAD
- Suicide risk: 4.1 times higher when there is no associated depression
- Suicide risk: 5,9 times greater when depression is associated

(Vasconcelos *et al*., 2015).

In the pathophysiology of anxiety disorders, there are biochemical components with the involvement of two neurotransmitters: serotonin 5-HT and GABA (gamma-amino butyric acid). Serotonin acts on a brain structure known as the amygdala, involved in emotional reactions and emotional learning, and in the dorsal periaqueductal gray matter, involved in defense behavior. Amygdala seems to act in the threat assessment and in the type of defense reaction to be done, while dorsal periaqueductal gray substance should be activated only in situations of imminent danger. Serotonin acts in regulating anxiety as an anxiogenic in the amygdala and as an anxiolytic in dorsal periaqueductal gray matter. Serotonin reuptake inhibiting drugs prolong the action of the neurotransmitter, probably causing an adaptive effect on the central nervous system. Gamma-amino butyric acid (GABA), the main inhibitory neurotransmitter in the central nervous system (CNS), has an anxiolytic effect probably due to the reduction in the activity of neuronal groups in the limbic system responsible for integrating defense reactions against loss or damage threats or reactions defenses caused by new situations. Some drugs, such as benzodiazepines, stimulate the action of GABA by suppressing neuronal activity in the response to stress (Konkewitz et al., 2010).

The treatment of generalized anxiety disorder involves a cognitive-behavioral and medication psychological therapeutic approach, with serotonin reuptake inhibiting drugs, tricyclic antidepressants or benzodiazepines for periods of less than 30 days (Associação Brasileira de Psiquiatria, 2008).

9. ANXIETY DISORDERS IN THE BIBLE

When we study mental disorders, we can better understand their causes, importance, pathophysiological bases and treatments. However, when it comes to pastors, we also need to turn to the Bible to identify God' servants who suffered from these diseases.

"That day, David fled from Saul and went to Achish king of Gath. But the servants of Achish said to him, "Isn't this David, the king of the land? Isn't he the one they sing about in their dances: "Saul has slain his thousands, and David his tens of thousands?" David took these words to heart and was very much afraid of Achish king of Gath. So he pretended to be insane in their presence; and while he was in their hands he acted like a madman, making marks on the doors of the gate and letting saliva run down his beard" (1 Samuel 21.10-13 – NIV).

"David left Gath and escaped to the cave of Adullam. When his brothers and his father's household heard about it, they went down to him there. All those who were in distress or in debt or discontented gathered around him, and he became their commander. About four hundred men were with him. From there David went to Mizpah in Moab and said to the king of Moab, "Would you let my father and mother come and stay with you **until I learn what God will do for me**?" (1 Samuel 22.1-3 - NIV).

David, the chief king of the Hebrews, is perhaps the prototype of the sufferer of mental disorders. These texts show that David was on the run from Saul, sentenced to death. David flees to Gate, which was one of the five Philistine principalities, enemies of Israel, thinking he would never be recognized. However, when he was recognized, he despaired, pretending to be crazy, and the Bible describes that David was "very afraid". In Hebrew, the expression used is "וַיִּרָא מְאֹד"(*Yir'ah Meod*). The word "וַיִּרָא" (*Yir'ah*) means "fear", "terror" (Strong Dictionary), while "מְאֹד" (*Meod*) can be translated as "greatness", "strength", "abundance" (Strong Dictionary) or, still, "excessively" (Brown-Driver-Briggs Dictionary). David was stricken with fear, excessive terror (anxiety disorder). David was suffering from generalized anxiety, so desperate that he ran away and hid in a cave. His parents came to help him, but the despair was so great that he left them with the king of Moab until "he knew what God would do to him", revealing feelings of hopelessness. This picture of mental stress, generalized anxiety and hopelessness blinded David's mind, understanding and faith. He had been anointed by the prophet Samuel as the future king of Israel, as determined by God, but he was suffering so much that he did not know what it would be like to forget God's promises for his life. Generalized anxiety makes us forget God's promises and provisions for our lives, producing hopelessness and predisposing us to depression, just as it was happening to David.

The apostle Paul also suffered from anxiety.

"Besides everything else, I face daily the **pressure of my concern** for all the churches" (2 Corinthians 11.28 – NIV).

Paul wrote to the Corinthian church and spoke about the struggles and difficulties he had been through, describing feelings of psychological suffering and anxiety. In Greek, the word used for "pressure of my concern" is "επισύστασίς" (*episustasis*), which means "a hostile group" or "gathering", "inciting a revolting gathering of people to riot", "running over someone" (Strong Dictionary). Paul describes an inner feeling as if there were a hostile crowd within him, as a psychological battle that slaughtered him. When he speaks of "concern", Paul uses the Greek word "μέριμνα" (*merimna*), which means "anxiety" (Strong Dictionary), describing not just any care or concern, but a feeling of anxiety. Paul had a concern of such magnitude that it caused intense psychological suffering that characterizes an anxiety disorder.

Jesus himself experienced a situation of extreme anxiety in Gethsemane.

"He withdrew about a stone's throw beyond them, knelt down and prayed, "Father, if you are willing, take this cup from me; yet not my will, but yours be done." An angel from heaven appeared to him and strengthened him. And **being in anguish, he prayed more earnestly, and his sweat was like drops of blood** falling to the ground" (Luke 22.41-44 – NIV).

Jesus was 100% God and 100% man, but he emptied himself of his condition as God and, as a man, suffered all the emotions suffered by human beings. Jesus, as God, knew exactly what was in store for him and that the pain would be so great that, as a man, he even asked the Father to, if possible, free him from sacrifice. The expectation and the certainty of suffering were terrifying and caused enormous anguish. In this anguish of expectation, Jesus, the man, lived a moment of extreme generalized anxiety. The anxiety was so great that Jesus presented an extremely rare phenomenon known as hematidrosis in which the human being exudes blood under conditions of extreme physical or emotional stress (Tshifularo, 2014).

We have a great reflection to make here: If Jesus suffered from extreme anxiety, why would not pastors be also subjected to anxiety disorders?

10. DEPRESSIVE DISORDERS

Depressive disorders are characterized by feelings of sadness, loss of interest or pleasure, guilt or low self-esteem, tiredness, difficulties in concentration, sleep or appetite disorders, recurring or long lasting, impairing the individual's ability to work, study and daily activities of life, which may lead to suicide, and include two main subcategories: major depressive disorder and dysthymia (WHO, 2017).

"Major depressive disorder represents the classic condition in this group of disorders. It is characterized by discrete episodes of at least 2 weeks' duration (although most episodes last considerably longer) involving clear-cut changes in affect, cognition, and neurovegetative functions and inter-episode remissions. A more chronic form of depression, persistent depressive disorder (dysthymia), can be diagnosed when the mood disturbance continues for at least 2 years in adults or 1 year in children". (DSM V, 2013).

Depressive disorders are different from bipolar disorders, which typically consist of episodes of mania and depression interspersed with periods of normal mood. In episodes of mania, the person behaves as if he were "the owner of the world" with exacerbated mood and increased energy, expansiveness, resulting in hyperactivity, loquacity, inflated self-esteem, feeling of greatness, pressure to speak, decreased need for sleep (DSM V, 2013; WHO, 2017). In depressive episodes, the person behaves as if he were "the garbage of the world". In mania, "buy the world", while in depression "surrender the soul and want the world to end".

Depressive disorders are the first cause of absence from work in the world (WHO, 2017), are more common in women (5.1%) than in men (3.6%) and have the following incidences:

- World: 4.4%
- United States of America, Estonia e Australia: 5.9%
- Brazil: 58%
- Portugal: 5.7% (WHO, 2017)
- Pastors: 9.1% or 154% higher than the general population (Duke Clergy Health Initiative, 2014)
- Suicide risk: 6.6 times larger than the general population in major depression
- Suicide risk: Risk 6.4 times larger than the general population in dysthymia (Vasconcelos *et al.*, 2015)
- Depressive pastors: Suicide risk 16 to 16.5 times higher than the general population

First-degree relatives have a 2 to 4 times greater risk of developing the disease in relation to the general population (DSM V, 2013), however the mode of transmission is not yet clear and studies of molecular genetics did not identified specific changes so far.

Studies on the pathophysiology of depression have focused on the role of neurotransmitters. The observations suggest that monoaminoxidase-inhibiting drugs (MAOIs) increase neuronal concentrations of norepinephrine and serotonin, decreasing their degradation by inhibiting the monoaminoxidase enzyme while tricyclic antidepressants increase the availability of these neurotransmitters by inhibiting the uptake in synaptic cleft. Serotonin, norepinephrine (or norepinephrine) and dopamine, together with acetylcholine, act in the modulation and integration of cortical and subcortical activities and are involved in the regulation of psychomotor activity, appetite, sleep and mood (Vallada Filho and Lafer, 1999).

Depressive disorders should be seen as multifactorial considering genetic, social, economic and biological aspects, and their treatment involves a cognitive-behavioral and problem-solving (in mild to moderate) psychotherapeutic approach, medication, with selective reuptake inhibitory drugs serotonin and tricyclic antidepressants and electroconvulsive therapy (ECT). Electroconvulsive therapy, popularly called "electroshock", despite being the most effective treatment available (80% to 90% response) and effective in half of patients who do not respond to medication, is not used as an initial treatment for depressive disorders due to side effects, need for general anesthesia and social stigma (Brazilian Association of Psychiatry, 2001).

11. DEPRESSIVE DISORDERS IN THE BIBLE

Just as we find several examples of anxiety disorders in the Bible, we can also find cases of servants of God suffering from depression.

David, due to his life history and trajectory of battles and wars, was always under high levels of stress that contributed to his psychological suffering.

"David **left Gath and escaped to the cave of Adullam**. When his brothers and his father's household heard about it, they went down to him there. All those who were in distress or in debt or discontented gathered around him, and he became their commander. About four hundred men were with him. From there David went to Mizpah in Moab and said to the king of Moab, "Would you let my father and mother come and stay with you **until I learn what God will do for me**?" (1 Samuel 22.1-3 - NIV).

David was suffering from generalized anxiety, running away from Saul who wanted to kill him, and had feelings of hopelessness with signs of depression (which occurs in 53.7% of people with GAD). He was so severe that he hid in a cave, seeking security and some psychological comfort in isolation and darkness. The depressed person, as a rule, assumes behavior of social isolation, does not seek or accept help and we can see this when his parents came to help him, but David left them with the king of Moab.

As hopelessness increases, depression deepens and thoughts of death arise.

"The cords of death entangled me; the torrents of destruction overwhelmed me. The cords of the grave coiled around me; the snares of death confronted me" (**Psalm 18.4-5 – NIV**)

David perfectly describes a severe and profound depressive condition, triggered by the constant stress he had always been subjected.

"Be merciful to me, LORD, for I am in distress; my eyes grow weak with sorrow, my soul and body with grief. My life is consumed by anguish and my years by groaning; my strength fails because of my affliction, and my bones grow weak. Because of all my enemies, I am the utter contempt of my neighbors and an object of dread to my closest friends— those who see me on the street flee from me. I am forgotten as though I were dead; I have become like broken pottery. For I hear many whispering, "Terror on every side!" They conspire against me and plot to take my life" (**Psalm 31.9-13 - NIV**).

Ruth's mother-in-law, Naomi, was another person who suffered from depression after the loss of her husband and children.

"When Naomi realized that Ruth was determined to go with her, she stopped urging her. So the two women went on until they came to Bethlehem. When they arrived in Bethlehem, the whole town was stirred because of them, and the women exclaimed, "Can this be **Naomi**?". "Don't call me **Naomi**" she told them. "Call me **Mara**, because the Almighty has made my life very bitter. I went away full, but the LORD has brought me back empty. Why call me Naomi? The LORD has afflicted me; the Almighty has brought misfortune upon me." **(Ruth 1.18-21 – NIV).**

After the death of her husband and children, Naomi returns to Bethlehem accompanied only by her daughter-in-law Ruth. "Naomi", in the Hebrew "נָעֳמִי" *(No'omiy)*, means "my delight". It derives from "נעם"*(No'am)*, which means "kindness", "kindness", "charm", "beauty", "favor" (Strong Dictionary). In turn, "Mara", in the Hebrew "מרה" *(Marah)*, means "bitter", "bitterness" (Strong Dictionary). Naomi felt so depressed that she wanted to be called as "bitterness".

Job was another person who suffered from depression.

"Do not mortals have hard service on earth? Are not their days like those of hired laborers? Like a slave longing for the evening shadows, or a hired laborer waiting to be paid, so I have been allotted months of futility, and nights of misery have been assigned to me. When I lie down I think, 'How long before I get up?' The night drags on, and I toss and turn until dawn. My body is clothed with worms and scabs, my skin is broken and festering. "My days are swifter than a weaver's shuttle, and they come to an end without hope. Remember, O God, that my life is but a breath; my eyes will never see happiness again. The eye that now sees me will see me no longer; you will look for me, but I will be no more. As a cloud vanishes and is gone, so one who goes down to the grave does not return. He will never come to his house again; his place will know him no more. "Therefore I will not keep silent; I will speak out in the anguish of my spirit, I will complain in the bitterness of my soul. Am I the sea, or the monster of the deep, that you put me under guard? When I think my bed will comfort me and my couch will ease my complaint, even then you frighten me with dreams and terrify me with visions, so that I prefer strangling and death, rather than this body of mine. I despise my life; I would not live forever. Let me alone; my days have no meaning" (Job 7.1-16 – NIV).

Job had lost his assets, his family, his health, and now he begins to lose his mental health. He shows signs of generalized anxiety with fear of even sleeping. The signs of depression start to become evident with insomnia, hopelessness, low self-esteem and ideas of contempt for life and death wishes. We know how God restored Job's life, but his mental health was greatly affected until healing process completion.

The prophet Elijah, much used by God to exhort the people, also suffered severely.

"Now Ahab told Jezebel everything Elijah had done and how he had killed all the prophets with the sword. So Jezebel sent a messenger to Elijah to say, "May the gods deal with me, be it ever so severely, if by this time tomorrow I do not make your life like that of one of them." Elijah **was afraid** and ran for his life. When he came to Beersheba in Judah, he left his servant there, while he himself went a day's journey into the wilderness. He came to a broom bush, sat down under it and prayed that he might die. "I have had enough, LORD," he said. "Take my life; I am no better than my ancestors." Then he lay down under the bush and fell asleep. All at once, an angel touched him and said, "Get up and eat." He looked around, and there by his head was some bread baked over hot coals, and a jar of water. He ate, drank, and then lay down again. The angel of the LORD came back a second time and touched him and said, "Get up and eat, for the journey is too much for you." So he got up and ate and drank. Strengthened by that food, he traveled forty days and forty nights until he reached Horeb, the mountain of God. There he went into a cave and spent the night. And the word of the LORD came to him: "What are you doing here, Elijah?" He replied, "I have been very zealous for the LORD God Almighty. The Israelites have rejected your covenant, torn down your altars, and put your prophets to death with the sword. I am the only one left, and now they are trying to kill me too." (1 Kings 19.1-10 – NIV).

Elijah witnessed and participated in God's great signs and miracles:

- Prophesied that it wouldn't rain for three years, and it didn't rain a drop
- He was fed by crows with bread and meat
- He lived in a widow's house and flour and oil multiplied through all the drought years
- Elijah resurrected the widow's son
- Elijah cried out and saw God pour fire and burn the holocaust that was completely drenched in water, before the prophets of Baal
- Elijah killed 450 Baal prophets
- He saw a small cloud, the size of a man's hand, turning into rain clouds and raining heavily

Even witnessing the power of God, Elijah suffered deeply from anxiety and depression. For what reasons did Elijah develop generalized anxiety and deep depression, despite knowing the power of God? Elijah had been under intense and continuous emotional stress for several years, and many events worked together to cause mental imbalance, such as:

- Elijah followed people's suffering and death during the drought
- The death of the son of Sarepta's widow shook him emotionally, even though he resurrected him
- He suffered from the murder of Israelites and their prophet friends who did not worship Baal and Asera

- The scenes of the deaths of Baal's prophets, bloody, violent and painful, ravaged his mind, like a "war trauma"
- Elijah knew Jezebel's wickedness

Going back to the scriptures, we can read the following:

"Elijah **was afraid** and ran for his life. When he came to Beersheba in Judah, he left his servant there" (1 Kings 19.3 – NVI).

In Hebrew the expression "was afraid", "וַיָּקָם" (*vayâqâm*), is in the third person singular of the verb "להה" (*lahahh*), according to the Hebrew Bible Stuttgartensia, and means "to fade" (Strong Dictionary); "Weaken", "dull", "lose the thread (cut)" (Hebrew Dictionary Pro online). Elijah was without strength, blunted behavior, typical depressive, as well as a knife that loses its cut, that is, he felt useless.

"while he himself **went a day's journey** into the wilderness" (1 Kings 19.4 – NIV)

"So he got up and ate and drank. Strengthened by that food, **he traveled forty days and forty nights** until he reached Horeb, the mountain of God" (1 Kings 19.8 – NIV)

In these texts, Elijah demonstrates a catatonic state, oblivious to the world around him, and walks off without stopping, similar to the race of three years, two months, fourteen days and sixteen hours of the character Forrest Gump, played by Tom Hanks in the film "Forrest Gump - The Story Teller, in 1994.

"while he himself went a day's journey into the wilderness. **He came to a broom bush, sat down under it and prayed that he might die**. "I have had enough, LORD," he said. "**Take my life**; I am no better than my ancestors" (1 Kings 19.4 – NIV).

"There **he went into a cave** and spent the night. And the word of the LORD came to him: "What are you doing here, Elijah?"" (1 Kings 19.9 – NIV)

When lying under the tree and entering the cave, Elijah was not simply looking for a shelter to protect himself from the weather, but was looking for a hiding place, for isolation, with feelings of self-deprecation and strong ideas of death.

12. BURNOUT SYNDROME

"Burnout syndrome" or "professional burn-out syndrome" or "feeling of being finished" is described as "extreme physical, mental and emotional exhaustion, resulting from prolonged exposure to situations of emotional and interpersonal stress in the professional or work environment". Burnout syndrome, or simply "burnout", was first described in 1974 by Herbert Freudenberger, German psychoanalyst, immigrant living in the United States, based on observations of its own behavior. Freudenberger used the expression "staff burnout" to describe a syndrome consisting of exhaustion, disillusionment and isolation in mental health workers (Trigo et al., 2007). In this situation, the person always very emotionally involved with his clients or work, suffers a continuous process of wear and tear until the moment when he loses energy and gives up to continue the activity, because the work loses its meaning, considering any effort as useless (Ministry of Health of Brazil, 2001).

Burnout is based on the following pillars:

- Emotional exhaustion: personal dimension in which negative feelings are directed at the person. They are feelings of emotional exhaustion and emotional emptying, feeling of exhaustion, lack of energy and emotional conditions to deal with routine work situations.

- Depersonalization: interpersonal dimension in which feelings turn to other people through negative feelings and attitudes, lack of empathy, sensitivity, indifference or excessive distance from people who should receive their services or care
- Decrease in personal involvement at work: organizational dimension when feelings turn against work, with feelings of decreased competence and success at work, directly affecting the form of service and contact with customers, patients and the company itself (Trigo et al., 2007; Portal da Educação, 2019).

Burnout is internationally recognized as an occupational risk for professional activities involving health care, education and assistance (Trigo et al., 2007). It is included in the 10th revision of the International Statistical Classification of Diseases and Health Problems or "International Classification of Diseases" (ICD-10), as "Z73.0 – State of vital exhaustion" (group "Z73 - Problems related to life-management difficulty"). In the 11th review (ICD-11), burnout is no longer considered a "medical condition" but is considered as an "occupational phenomenon", in the chapter 24 "Factors influencing health status or contact with health services", encoded as "QD85 – Problems associated with employment or unemployment".

According to the 11th revision of the International Statistical Classification of Diseases and Health Problems (ICD-11), "burn-out is a syndrome conceptualized as resulting from chronic workplace stress that has not been successfully managed. It is characterized by three dimensions:

- Feelings of energy depletion or exhaustion;
- Increased mental distance from one's job, or feelings of negativism or cynicism related to one's job; and
- A sense of ineffectiveness and lack of accomplishment.

Burn-out refers specifically to phenomena in the occupational context and should not be applied to describe experiences in other areas of life". (ICD-11 - WHO, 2019).

Epidemiologically, the establishment of risk factors for burnout involves the organization, the individual, work and society.

- Organization: Bureaucracy (excess of norms), lack of autonomy (inability to make decisions without consulting or obtaining authorization), rigid institutional rules that prevent workers from achieving autonomy and feeling in control of their tasks, frequent organizational changes (frequent changes rules and norms), lack of trust, respect and consideration among team members, inefficient communication causing distortions and slowness in the dissemination of information, inability to ascend in the career and improve their remuneration and recognition, physical environment and their risks, including heat, cold and excessive noise or insufficient lighting, poor hygiene, high toxic and even life risk, accumulation of tasks, living with colleagues affected by the syndrome

- Individual: Related to personality characteristics and associated with a greater predisposition. Competitive, hardworking, impatient individuals with an excessive need to control situations that show less tolerance for frustration; with a high degree of empathy; pessimists who suffer in anticipation of the possibility of failure; perfectionists, overly demanding of themselves and like others and who do not tolerate mistakes; that they are more subject to emotional exhaustion while men suffer more from depersonalization; higher educational level.

- Work: Overload or excessive quality of demands beyond capacity due to personal technical deficiency, insufficient time or lack of infrastructure; small participation in decisions about organizational changes; poor organizational support; intensity or proximity in the relations with the people to whom it must attend.

- Society: Lack of social and family support to share the anxieties; difficulty in maintaining the social status associated with the profession due to low pay or the inability to manage personal resources using overtime or additional jobs, causing physical exhaustion and dissatisfaction (Trigo et al., 2007).

The feeling of low professional achievement is the most important factor in triggering burnout for the evaluated pastors, while the literature points to emotional exhaustion and depersonalization as the main factors in the general population. The main elements pointed out were physical tiredness, emotional involvement with members, superficiality in the relationship with peers, the demand for results, the complexity of pastoral work and the lack of recognition at work (Santos and Honório, 2014). Despite the various roles and functions performed and the difficulties in dealing with complex interpersonal relationships, the incidence of burnout in pastors, apparently, is similar to other assistance activities, probably because they are able to cope well with challenges and maintain optimism because they consider that the call to the ministry is profoundly significant (Duke Clergy Health Initiative, 2014).

Burnout is one of the main diseases in Europe and the United States of America, alongside diabetes and cardiovascular diseases (Akerstedt, 2004; Weber & Jackel-Reinhardt, 2000), with an estimated annual cost of more than 150 billion American dollars (Donatelle & Hawkings, 1989). It is responsible for an increase in medical costs between 46% to 147%, when associated with depression (Goetzel et al., 1998) and has the following incidences:

- General population: 4.2% (Houtman et al., 1998)
- United States of America: More than 40% in doctors (Henderson, 1984)
- Brazil: 26% among teachers (Codo, 1999)
- Pastors: Similar to other professions (Duke Clergy Health Initiative, 2014)

So far, there is no clear established neuroendocrine involvement.

Burnout treatment is multifaceted, encompassing psychotherapy, medications and psychosocial interventions. Even with drug treatment, psychotherapy is always indicated as a form of emotional support to enable restructuring of thought and reinsertion into life and work. Drug treatment results, using antidepressants, are observed two to four weeks after the start of medication. Eventually, benzodiazepine anxilolytics may be associated, for short periods, to control anxiety and insomnia at the beginning of treatment. Psychosocial interventions with removal from work may be necessary due to medical advice for treatment.

Prevention probably is the best strategy to combat burnout with changes in organizational culture, restrictions on overwork, establishment of collective goals including individual well-being, multidisciplinary teams trained to provide emotional support and early detection of signs of burn-out (Health Ministry of Brazil, 2001).

In the Old Testament Jethro, Moses' father-in-law, observes the son-in-law's daily routine, realizes his exhaustion in serving people and guides for preventive measures against burnout:

"The next day Moses took his seat to serve as judge for the people, and they stood around him from morning till evening. When his father-in-law saw all that Moses was doing for the people, he said, "What is this you are doing for the people? Why do you alone sit as judge, while all these people stand around you from morning till evening?" Moses answered him, "Because the people come to me to seek God's will. Whenever they have a dispute, it is brought to me, and I decide between the parties and inform them of God's decrees and instructions." Moses' father-in-law replied, "What you are doing is not good. You and these people who come to you will only wear yourselves out. The work is too heavy for you; you cannot handle it alone. Listen now to me and I will give you some advice, and may God be with you. You must be the people's representative before God and bring their disputes to him. Teach them his decrees and instructions, and show them the way they are to live and how they are to behave. But select capable men from all the people, men who fear God, trustworthy men who hate dishonest gain, and appoint them as officials over thousands, hundreds, fifties and tens. Have them serve as judges for the people at all times, but have them bring every difficult case to you; the simple cases they can decide themselves. That will make your load lighter, because they will share it with you. If you do this and God so commands, you will be able to stand the strain, and all these people will go home satisfied." **(Exodus 18.13-23 - NIV).**

13. BURNOUT SYNDROME IN THE BIBLE

Jethro instructed his son-in-law Moses to prevent burnout syndrome, but in the Bible, we find people suffering from this disorder.

Jeremiah is one of the examples of people suffering from burnout:

"You deceived me, LORD, and I was deceived; you overpowered me and prevailed. I am ridiculed all day long; everyone mocks me. Whenever I speak, I cry out proclaiming violence and destruction. So the word of the LORD has brought me insult and reproach all day long. But if I say, "I will not mention his word or speak anymore in his name," his word is in my heart like a fire, a fire shut up in my bones. I am weary of holding it in; indeed, I cannot. I hear many whispering, "Terror on every side! Denounce him! Let's denounce him!" All my friends are waiting for me to slip, saying, "Perhaps he will be deceived; then we will prevail over him and take our revenge on him." But the LORD is with me like a mighty warrior; so my persecutors will stumble and not prevail. They will fail and be thoroughly disgraced; their dishonor will never be forgotten. LORD Almighty, you who examine the righteous and probe the heart and mind, let me see your vengeance on them, for to you I have committed my cause. Sing to the LORD! Give praise to the LORD! He rescues the life of the needy from the hands of the wicked. Cursed be the day I was born! May the day my mother bore me not be blessed! Cursed be the man who brought my father the news, who made him very glad, saying, "A child is born to you—a son!" May that man be like the towns the LORD overthrew without pity. May he hear wailing in the morning, a battle cry at noon. For he did not kill me in the womb, with my mother as my grave, her womb enlarged forever. Why did I ever come out of the womb to see trouble and sorrow and to end my days in shame?" (Jeremiah 20.7-18 – NIV).

    Jeremiah had a prophetic ministry for about 40 years, bringing harsh words of exhortation to the people of Israel. Because of the harsh prophecies, Jeremiah was mocked and even physically assaulted. In addition to the various types of physical and moral aggression, the weight of the prophecies also affected their emotions and affected their psychological health. While trying to please and serve God, Jeremiah suffered at the hands of men, felt "deceived" by God and lived a great inner conflict, without strength and without courage to continue his prophetic ministry. The stress and emotional imbalance were so intense that Jeremiah cursed his mother for giving birth to him, his father and even the person who delivered her. Jeremiah was in severe burnout, with signs of anxiety and depression, resulting from chronic exposure to stress.

    Looking closely at the situation that Jeremiah was experiencing, it is easy to understand that pastors are subject to exhaustion, by understanding that the very nature of their profession and the characteristics of the activity predispose the syndrome.

14. SUICIDE

Suicide, in itself, is not considered as a mental disorder, but as a consequence of it. It takes great importance because incidence has been increased among pastors, which did not occur a few decades ago. The expected death, whether natural due to old age or illness, is a painful event, tragic deaths (accidents, homicides, etc.) are traumatic, but suicide deaths, in addition to the pain of loss and trauma of the event, carry countless others. Feelings, such as the search for an answer, often not found, even guilt for not being able to perceive the risk, or for avoiding the suicide of the intimate person. Estimates indicate that, in 2012, there were about 804,000 suicides in the world, which means a rate of 11.4 per 100,000 people, and rates are higher in men (15.0) than in women (8.0). Women attempt suicide more than men, but with less lethal success. There is no simple answer to suicide, but social, cultural and psychological factors, among others, can interact as predisposing factors for suicidal behavior (WHO, 2014).

From a psychological point of view, there is an increased risk of suicide by up to 6.6 times in patients suffering from major depression and 4.1 times in individuals with generalized anxiety disorder without associated depression (Vasconcelos et al., 2015). The subject assumes greater importance among pastors, given the higher incidence of depressive conditions in these professional groups (Duke Clergy Health Initiative, 2014).

The best approach in combating suicide is, without a doubt, prevention, mainly by identifying suicidal risk behaviors, such as previous suicide attempts, psychological disorders (present in 90% of people who die by suicide), alcohol abuse and drugs, feelings of hopelessness, family history of suicide, financial and professional difficulties (unemployment) and chronic illnesses or pain. There is a myth that those who really want to commit suicide do not warn, but verbal or behavioral warning signs precede most cases and should not be overlooked or ignored. Not every suicide is determined to die, but they have mixed feelings about continuing to live or die (WHO, 2014). In this context, pastors face greater difficulties because they do not have a personal support network, or do not feel safe to share their feelings, due to fear of judgments about their spirituality and ability to lead the church. Suicide prevention requires vision, planning and establishing strategies that require scientific and practical knowledge, emotional support and social strategy (WHO, 2014), and churches and denominations need to break paradigms and prejudices to help the pastor restore his emotional balance and advance life and even in ministry.

15. PROVISIONS FROM GOD

All human beings can suffer from illnesses, whether physical, mental or spiritual, and the pastor would not be an exception. Strenuous workload and emotional exhaustion are important factors that affect the health of the pastor as a whole. The theological approach based on the Gospel of John recognizes afflictions, but presents in a masterful way the loving Father who gave his only begotten son for the redemption of man and the Holy Spirit to reveal the mysteries of his kingdom.

"I have told you these things, so that in me you may have peace. In this world you will have **TROUBLE**. But take heart! I have overcome the world" **(John 16.33 - NIV)**

When Jesus refers to the "troubles" (in Greek: "θλιψις" - *thlipsis*) suffered by the human being, he demonstrates to know perfectly the amplitude of the situations and the suffering caused by them, as if the person were "crushed, pressed like grapes in the winepress". Metaphorically, Jesus spoke about the feeling of destruction and inner death brought about by these extreme situations. Jesus does not promise the apostles a life without mishaps and bad weather, but, on the contrary, he warns that they would be persecuted and hated, however, he also ensures that the Father would provide the means to overcome the hardships of life.

"No **temptation** has overtaken you except what is common to mankind. And God is faithful; he will not let you be tempted beyond what you can bear. But when you are tempted, he will also provide a way out so that you can endure it" (1 Corinthians 10.13 - NIV).

In Greek, the word "πειρασμος" (*peirasmos*) is used, which can be translated not only by "temptation", "trial or ordeal" or "seduction to sin", but also by "adversity", "trouble" or "annoyance" (Dictionary Strong).

Mental health disorders are well described in the medical literature, defining the diagnosis, neuroendocrine involvement, pathophysiology and treatment. This scientific knowledge must be used and understood as a providence from God for the human being, as well as a father who spares no effort to his children's good.

God can provide the means for the restoration of people, by his unique, exclusive and indisputable will. According to his incomprehensible wisdom, God can heal some by supernatural action, others by natural means (people, medicines) while others will not receive physical healing, but the opportunity to recognize the greatness of his love and mercy in the revelation of Christ's redemptive sacrifice that makes us his children. God in his omniscience deeply knows his creation (limitations, desires, wants, difficulties) and, because of his great love, takes care of his children:

"Just as the providence of God in general extends to every creature, so, in a very special way it takes care of his church and orders all things for its good" (The Westminster Confession of Faith, Chapter V, Item VII).

Mental health problems are of great importance not only due to high incidence rates, but also due to difficulties in seeking help and treatment, mainly due to the lack of emotional support mechanisms established by churches or denominations aimed at the pastor and his family and prejudice regarding this group of disorders. The "afflictions" of life can negatively affect the physical and mental health of human beings, and pastors and religious ministers are not free to be affected by them. The big question is management, "how to deal" with these health problems. The treatment of these conditions can involve several aspects, according to the medical literature: changes in lifestyle, personal support, psychotherapy and medication:

1. Changes in lifestyle: changes in social, work and food habits
2. Personal support: Moral, motivational support, through the network of relationships of friends, groups, communities, church, without necessarily technical or professional training in the health area
3. Psychotherapy: Professional assistance with application of knowledge of Psychology, Psychiatry and Psychopathology
4. Drug treatment: Use of drugs with chemical properties to restore neuroendocrine balance

Medical and psychological literature has also studied the importance and impact of spirituality in the treatment of mental health problems, recognizing lower probabilities of mental illness and better results in the treatment of patients who exercise their faith (Lotufo Neto, 1997; Vollet & Wiggers, 2019), showing that the relationship with God is one of the "relieves", "escapes" or one of the "ways out to endure them", given by the Father.

Thus, all approaches in the treatment of mental disorders, from supernatural healing to the use of medications, should be considered as provisions from God for his children, without prejudice or restrictions.

16. THE DIVINE RESTORATION

The first way out provided by God is the divine action itself through relationship with him. There is no doubt, for those who know the Bible, that David suffered countless afflictions, both from persecutions and trauma of battles and from inner conflicts. David's life was extremely tense, living constantly under the expectation of the unexpected, of imminent danger, often not feeling physical security even in places where he sought refuge (1 Samuel 21.10-13). Such was the situation that David sought physical refuge in hiding places in the desert, to which other people, equally afflicted, also resorted (1 Samuel 22: 1-2). However, David sought and recognized in God the source of all deliverance and relief from afflictions:

"You, LORD, keep my lamp burning; my God turns **my darkness** into light. With your help I can advance against a troop; with my God I can scale a wall. As for God, his way is perfect: The LORD's word is flawless; he shields all who take refuge in him. For who is God besides the LORD? And who is the Rock except our God? It is God who arms me with strength and keeps my way secure" (Psalm 18.28-32 - NIV).

David recognizes his afflictions and his feelings of abandonment and hopelessness, feeling immersed in darkness. More than purely a feeling of "anxiety", David demonstrated to live a "generalized anxiety disorder" and a depressive condition often associated with it (Gavin et al., 2015).

The description of the feeling of being in darkness ("my darkness") shows the deep depressive state in which David was immersed. David is conscious of his condition, but seeks and recognizes in the Lord's mercy restoration and comfort in adversity. In moments of deep anguish, he cries out to God in prayer:

"Listen to my prayer, O God, do not ignore my plea; hear me and answer me. My thoughts trouble me and I am distraught because of what my enemy is saying, because of the threats of the wicked; for they bring down suffering on me and assail me in their anger. My heart is in anguish within me; the terrors of death have fallen on me. Fear and trembling have beset me; horror has overwhelmed me. I said, "Oh, that I had the wings of a dove! I would fly away and be at rest. I would flee far away and stay in the desert; I would hurry to my place of shelter, far from the tempest and storm" (Psalm 55.1-8 - NVI).

Elements of anxiety disorder and major depression are observed, but David cries out to the Father in prayer and acknowledges the help:

"Cast your cares on the LORD and he will sustain you; he will never let the righteous be shaken" (Psalm 55.22 - NIV).

Paul was another servant of the Lord who suffered persecution and situations of extreme stress, recognizing, however, the importance of an intimate relationship with God to overcome afflictions. Paul directs to raise all concerns about the Lord by developing a life of prayer:

"And pray in the Spirit on all occasions with all kinds of prayers and requests. With this in mind, be alert and always keep on praying for all the Lord's people" (Ephesians 6.18 - NIV).

Paul insists on the importance of prayer, taking time to pray and being intimate with God. Intimacy produces confidence and the certainty of support. Only by developing intimacy with God is it possible to know and recognize God as a kind, loving and merciful father, in whom one can trust and deposit all needs, with the conviction that the best will be done, because God is in control.

Another way to overcome afflictions, in addition to prayer, is to occupy the mind with good and true things through knowledge and meditation on the Word of God:

"Blessed is the one who does not walk in step with the wicked or stand in the way that sinners take or sit in the company of mockers, but whose delight is in the law of the LORD, and who meditates on his law day and night" (Psalm 1.1-2 - NIV).

Knowledge of God is essential for trusting Him, and reading, knowledge and meditation on the Word are essential for the renewal of the mind, as if, metaphorically, the "formatting of the Hard Disk is made to remove viruses, malware, the" trash", and insert new, healthy and reliable information:

"Do not conform to the pattern of this world, but be transformed by the renewing of your mind. Then you will be able to test and approve what God's will is, his good, pleasing and perfect will" (Romans 12.2 - NIV).

Only by renewing the mind, the way of thinking, through meditation on the Word of God and the life of prayer, one can practice and live the truths of the Gospel and truly surrender life, afflictions, needs and hope in God:

"and to know this love that surpasses knowledge, that you may be filled to the measure of all the fullness of God. Now to him who is able to do immeasurably more than all we ask or imagine, according to his power that is at work within us" (Ephesians 3.19-20 - NIV).

17. LIFESTYLE CHANGES

Pastors and religious ministers' professional activities are extremely complex and intense, imposing a routine of life, usually, unruly, with regard to schedules, food, rest, vacations, leisure, coexistence and conjugal relationship and with the children. Often, church members see the pastor as a servant who should be available at any time and need. This level of demand and external expectations instills in the pastor the feeling of responsibility in meeting these demands in the best possible way. Often assuming a load of tasks impossible to be fulfilled generates high levels of stress, anxiety, frustration and physical and emotional exhaustion. Lifestyle changes or adaptations, including diet, are an important aspect in preventing and treating physical and mental health problems. The separation of time for rest is fundamental for the repair of vigor, so important that God himself rested and ordered the man to do the same:

"By the seventh day God had finished the work he had been doing; so on the seventh day he rested from all his work. Then God blessed the seventh day and made it holy, because on it he rested from all the work of creating that he had done" (Genesis 2.2-3 - NIV)

"For six days work is to be done, but the seventh day is a day of sabbath rest, holy to the LORD. Whoever does any work on the Sabbath day is to be put to death" (Exodus 31.15 – INV).

Adequate time management, in order to organize activities and commitments, is extremely important to fulfil effectively and efficiently tasks and commitments, without wasting time, efforts and resources. Paul instructs to use time wisely, prioritizing the most important things:

"Be very careful, then, how you live, not as unwise but as wise, **making the most of every opportunity**, because the days are evil" (Ephesians 5.15-16 - NIV).

"**15**. βλεπετε ουν πως ακριβως περιπατειτε μη ως ασοφοι αλλ ως σοφοι **16**. **εξαγοραζομενοι** τον καιρον οτι αι ημεραι πονηραι εισιν"

When Paul recommends "seizing" opportunities, or "**making the most of every opportunity**", he uses the verb "**εξαγοραζω**" (*exagorazo*) which means to rescue; buy for yourself, use every opportunity to do good in a wise and sacred way, so that zeal and goodness are, so to speak, the money of the purchase with which we save our time (Strong's Dictionary). In Greek, "**εξαγοραζω**" (*exagorazo*) and "**αγοραζω**" (*agorazo*) were words used in the slave markets and both meant "to buy". However, "αγοραζω" (*agorazo*) was used when the slave was purchased to be resold, while "εξαγοραζω" (*exagorazo*) indicates that the slave was being purchased as permanent possession. Thus, Paul guided the wise use of his own time, both in prioritizing activities and in the correct allocation of time, for work, rest, leisure, socialization and attention to family needs and relationships, as determined by the Old Testament:

"There is a time for everything, and a season for every activity under the heavens: a time to be born and a time to die, a time to plant and a time to uproot, a time to kill and a time to heal, a time to tear down and a time to build, a time to weep and a time to laugh, a time to mourn and a time to dance, a time to scatter stones and a time to gather them, a time to embrace and a time to refrain from embracing, a time to search and a time to give up, a time to keep and a time to throw away, a time to tear and a time to mend, a time to be silent and a time to speak, a time to love and a time to hate, a time for war and a time for peace" (Ecclesiastes 3.1-8 - NIV).

Another important aspect is the care with the correct diet to preserve physical health. In time management, it is important to establish an adequate meal schedule, as well as having healthy eating habits

18. PERSONAL SUPPORT

Moral and motivational assistance, through the network of relationships of friends, groups, communities, church, without necessarily technical or professional training in the health field, also presents itself as one of the forms of support to alleviate suffering and treatment of mental health problems. A classic example takes place when Paul was imprisoned in Rome and writes to Timothy, revealing that he feels abandoned by his brothers and the importance of the moral support he received from Onesíforo and his family:

"You know that everyone in the province of Asia has deserted me, including Phygelus and Hermogenes. May the Lord show mercy to the household of Onesiphorus, because he often refreshed me and was not ashamed of my chains. On the contrary, when he was in Rome, he searched hard for me until he found me" (2 Timothy 1.15-17 - INV).

Furthermore, Paul demonstrated feeling alone and his need for company and support:

"Do your best to come to me quickly, for Demas, because he loved this world, has deserted me and has gone to Thessalonica. Crescens has gone to Galatia, and Titus to Dalmatia. Only Luke is with me. Get Mark and bring him with you, because he is helpful to me in my ministry" (2 Timothy 4.9-11 - INV).

Jesus himself needed the support of his disciples. In Gethsemane, Jesus, overcome with such intense pain, sadness and anguish, Christ asked the support of his apostles and was upset because he did not receive the support he needed:

"Then Jesus went with his disciples to a place called Gethsemane, and he said to them, "Sit here while I go over there and pray." He took Peter and the two sons of Zebedee along with him, and he began to be sorrowful and troubled. Then he said to them, "My soul is overwhelmed with sorrow to the point of death. Stay here and keep watch with me." Going a little farther, he fell with his face to the ground and prayed, "My Father, if it is possible, may this cup be taken from me. Yet not as I will, but as you will." Then he returned to his disciples and found them sleeping. "Couldn't you men keep watch with me for one hour?" he asked Peter. "Watch and pray so that you will not fall into temptation. The spirit is willing, but the flesh is weak." He went away a second time and prayed, "My Father, if it is not possible for this cup to be taken away unless I drink it, may your will be done." When he came back, he again found them sleeping, because their eyes were heavy. So he left them and went away once more and prayed the third time, saying the same thing. Then he returned to the disciples and said to them, "Are you still sleeping and resting? Look, the hour has come, and the Son of Man is delivered into the hands of sinners. Rise! Let us go! Here comes my betrayer!" (Mathew 26.36-46 – NIV).

19. PROFISSIONAL ASSISTANCE

Christians easily accept the three previous approaches, however, in some cases they are not enough to restore mental health balance, requiring professional intervention and use of knowledge from Psychology, Psychiatry and Psychopathology. Here lies a great difficulty in the care and treatment of mental health problems. There are still many prejudices and misconceptions about psychological disorders, which associate them with sin and demonic influences or possessions. This inhibits a large part of pastors and religious ministers from seeking this type of assistance, either by this way of thinking or by fear of damage to their ministerial life due to the judgment made by the people. This association between illness and sin can generate guilt in people, when, in fact, the causes are different from it.

"As he went along, he saw a man blind from birth. His disciples asked him, "Rabbi, who sinned, this man or his parents, that he was born blind?". "Neither this man nor his parents sinned," said Jesus, "but this happened so that the works of God might be displayed in him" (John 9.1-3 - NIV).

The concept that mental disorders are due exclusively to demonic influences or possessions disregards the fact that, in accepting Jesus as lord and savior of his life, the Christian receives the Holy Spirit:

"But if Christ is in you, then even though your body is subject to death because of sin, the Spirit gives life because of righteousness. And if the Spirit of him who raised Jesus from the dead is living in you, he who raised Christ from the dead will also give life to your mortal bodies because of his Spirit who lives in you" (Romans 8.10-11 - NIV).

The true Christian cannot be possessed by demons, for his body is the temple of the Holy Spirit and, as such, cannot be shared with darkness:

"Do you not know that your bodies are temples of the Holy Spirit, who is in you, whom you have received from God? You are not your own, you were bought at a price. Therefore honor God with your bodies" (1 Corinthians 6.19-20 - NIV).

Support and assistance from other people undoubtedly have their value, however, often the severity of mental health problems and theoretical ignorance about the basis of human behavior, psychopathology and the lack of adequate education and training limit the effectiveness in restoring the individual's psychological balance. The complexity of the human mind is so great that inner conflicts can paralyze the individual. Paul revealed the conflicts he experienced as consequence of his past:

"I do not understand what I do. For what I want to do I do not do, but what I hate I do. And if I do what I do not want to do, I agree that the law is good. As it is, it is no longer I myself who do it, but it is sin living in me. For I know that good itself does not dwell in me, that is, in my sinful nature. For I have the desire to do what is good, but I cannot carry it out. For I do not do the good I want to do, but the evil I do not want to do, his I keep on doing. Now if I do what I do not want to do, it is no longer I who do it, but it is sin living in me that does it. So I find this law at work: Although I want to do good, evil is right there with me. For in my inner being I delight in God's law; but I see another law at work in me, waging war against the law of my mind and making me a prisoner of the law of sin at work within me. What a wretched man I am! Who will rescue me from this body that is subject to death? Thanks be to God, who delivers me through Jesus Christ our Lord! So then, I myself in my mind am a slave to God's law, but in my sinful nature a slave to the law of sin" (Romans 7.15-25 – NIV).

Paul was not possessed by demons, for sure, but he was experiencing an inner conflict, as well as nowadays many pastors, religious ministers, lay and Christian workers, also are experiencing different levels of psychological suffering. This fact has favored and encouraged academic training for counseling professionals, psychotherapy and other scientifically based therapies, and adequate respect for the Christian faith. In Brazil, for example, there is an association of Christian psychiatrists and psychologists with the purpose of developing creative studies on the relations of the psychological sciences and Hebrew-Christian theology and philosophy (www.cppc.org.br). In the United States of America, there are many Christian counselors and therapists as well.

20. DRUG THERAPY

If the professional psychological or psychiatric counseling approach encounters resistance based on misconceptions about mental disorders, drug treatment carries with it the subjective concepts of "madness", "insanity", not only among Christians, but also in society as a whole. This misconception is based upon the treatment administered to patients in the not-too-distant past, due to the lack of knowledge about pathophysiology, biochemistry and the small range of drugs available. Currently, the role of neurotransmitters in the most diverse psychiatric disorders is well established, especially the involvement of serotonin, dopamine and norepinephrine, which can be affected by numerous situations, including continuous and prolonged exposure to stress, eating habits, nutritional deficiencies (tryptophan, amino acid precursor of serotonin, for example), genetic factors and the normal aging process. This knowledge allowed the development of drugs with better results and less adverse effects for the treatment of these diseases.

God can actually perform miraculous healings:

"Is anyone among you sick? Let them call the elders of the church to pray over them and anoint them with oil in the name of the Lord. And the prayer offered in faith will make the sick person well; the Lord will raise them up. If they have sinned, they will be forgiven" (James 5.14-15 - NIV).

The use of medicines for diseases treatment and healing, however, does not mean lack of faith, since we know that, in his sovereignty, God can heal some and not others, according to his purposes:

"God uses ordinary means to work out his providence day by day. But, as he pleases, he may work without, beyond, or contrary to these means" (The Westminster Confession of Faith, Chapter V, Item III).

The apostle Paul suffered from an evil, which he regarded as "a thorn in the flesh" which, however much he asked, did not have a cure, but he understood that there was a purpose of God for this to happen:

"or because of these surpassingly great revelations. Therefore, in order to keep me from becoming conceited, I was given a thorn in my flesh, a messenger of Satan, to torment me. Three times I pleaded with the Lord to take it away from me. But he said to me, "My grace is sufficient for you, for my power is made perfect in weakness." Therefore I will boast all the more gladly about my weaknesses, so that Christ's power may rest on me" (2 Corinthians 12.7-9 – NIV).

Paul, however, also understood and recognized that diseases could be treated with medicines, so much so that recommends to Timothy the therapeutic use of wine:

"Stop drinking only water, and use a little wine because of your stomach and your frequent illnesses" (1 Timothy 5.23 - NIV).

Jesus, even if metaphorically, alludes to the need for medical treatment for the sick:

"While Jesus was having dinner at Matthew's house, many tax collectors and sinners came and ate with him and his disciples. When the Pharisees saw this, they asked his disciples, "Why does your teacher eat with tax collectors and sinners?" On hearing this, Jesus said, "It is not the healthy who need a doctor, but the sick" (Mathew 9.10-12 - NIV).

In the parable of the Good Samaritan, Jesus mentions the use of medicines to treat wounds:

"He went to him and bandaged his wounds, pouring on oil and wine. Then he put the man on his own donkey, brought him to an inn and took care of him" (Luke 10.34 - NIV).

In the Old Testament, there is also mention of medicines and doctors:

"Fruit trees of all kinds will grow on both banks of the river. Their leaves will not wither, nor will their fruit fail. Every month they will bear fruit, because the water from the sanctuary flows to them. Their fruit will serve for food and their leaves for healing" (Ezekiel 47.12 - NIV)

"Is there no balm in Gilead? Is there no physician there? Why then is there no healing for the wound of my people?" (Jeremiah 8.12 - NIV).

As it can be concluded, mental health disorders have organic, biochemical and/or neuroendocrine components, and may require adequate drug treatment to restore the individual's health balance, enabling a return to normal personal life, healthy family and social lives and the perform ministerial activities productively. There is no solid biblical argument against the use of drug therapy for the treatment of mental disorders as well for any other disease.

21. FINAL CONSIDERATIONS

People experience various situations in their daily routines of life, experiencing all kinds of feelings and experiences that produce moments of happiness and well-being, but also of sadness, suffering and physical, mental and spiritual pain. Pastors and religious ministers could not be different from other people. Pastoral activity requires dedication and personal, family and social renunciations to meet the expectations and needs of the church and its members, often in an intensity far superior to what can be endured. The demands placed on the pastor, whether in the administration and growth of the church or in a preaching that pleases and meets the wishes of members, in association to other aspects, such as the remuneration often insufficient for exclusive dedication to the ministry, absence of well-defined working hours requiring full availability to meet the needs of the church and its members, lack of a support network to meet the needs of the pastor and his family, the competitive relationship with other pastors, the feeling of loneliness in the ministry, among others, are factors that produce stress ("stressors") at varying levels. The intensity and constancy of these stressors over the pastor can impact physical and mental health, triggering anxiety disorders, depression, burn-out and even though suicide at rates higher than those observed in the general population, requiring appropriate treatment. However, there are several obstacles for the pastor to seek and find this treatment, being prejudice related to mental disorders, probably, the main one.

The lack of theoretical knowledge and understanding about these disorders, often attributed to sin, lack of faith, weak spirituality and madness, are undoubtedly important barriers that need to be broken when seeking treatment. The church, and the pastor himself, must recognize mental disorders as diseases like any other and that God, in his infinite wisdom, mercy and love, provides all the means for a proper treatment, health restoration, emotional and spiritual balance, either through supernatural healing or through trained people, used by the almighty Father to indicate the use of appropriate medicines. In addition, mental disorders must be treated in their causes in a prophylactic way. Churches and religious denominations must set up programs, norms or policies to support, prevent and treat their pastors' physical and mental health, through the establishment of an adequate work regime, observing weekly rest periods and paid vacations, adequate remuneration or conditions to meet the pastor and his family's basic needs, availability of a structure or support network for care and attention to physical and mental health, among other measures, in order to preserve the pastor's health so that the health of the church itself is preserved.

ABOUT THE AUTHOR

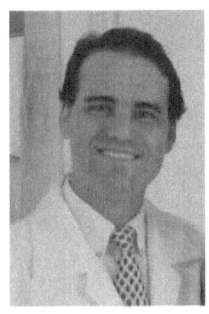

Delcio Torres Amorim Junior, graduated in Agronomy from the Londrina State University (www.uel.br), in 1986, worked in multinational companies. Graduated in Medicine from the Londrina State University (www.uel.br), in 1996, and medical residency in General Surgery from the São Paulo Pontifical Catholic University (www.pucsp.br), receiving the title of specialist in General Surgery (1998). Former medical officer in the Brazilian Air Force, practiced medicine in important hospitals in São Paulo. Master in Business Administration from Fundação Getúlio Vargas (www.fgv.br), in 2004. Worked in the management areas of large companies operating health plans in São Paulo. Completed a high school degree in Theology at the Hosanna Theological Seminary (1992) and a Master's in Theology at the Philadelphia University Center – UniFil (www.unifil.br), in 2019. Presbyterian pastor, collaborating at Central Presbyterian Church in Londrina, Brazil (www.igrejacentral.com.br). Professor in the postgraduate course in psychoanalysis and member of the academic and scientific board at the International Institute of Psychoanalysis.

Married to Sonne Keopis, a real estate, they have two children (Philip and Isabella). Creator and coordinator of "The Potter's House", a comprehensive health care program for pastors and their families. Currently practices medicine in Londrina (Brazil).

Contact: drdelcio@hotmail.com

REFERENCES

ASSOCIAÇÃO AMERICANA DE PSIQUIATRIA (APA). DSM IV - Manual Diagnóstico e Estatístico para Transtornos Mentais, 4ª versão. Washington (DC): American Psychiatric Press; 1994.

ASSOCIAÇÃO AMERICANA DE PSIQUIATRIA (APA). DSM V - Manual Diagnóstico e Estatístico para Transtornos Mentais, 5ª versão. Tradução de Maria Inês Corrêa Nascimento et al. Porto Alegre. Artmed. 2014. Available at http:// www.niip.com.br/wp-content/uploads/2018/06/ Manual- Diagnosico- e- Estatistico- de- Transtornos- Mentais- DSM-5-1-pdf.pdf. Access in 06/19/2019.

ASSOCIAÇÃO BRASILEIRA DE PSIQUIATRIA. Diagnóstico e tratamento da depressão. Brasil. 2001. Available at https:// diretrizes. amb. org.br/ BibliotecaAntiga/ depressao.pdf. Access in 06/28/2019.

ASSOCIAÇÃO BRASILEIRA DE PSIQUIATRIA. Transtornos de ansiedade: Diagnóstico e tratamento. Brasil. 2008. Available at https:// diretrizes. amb. org.br/ BibliotecaAntiga/ transtornos- de- ansiedade- diagnostico- e-tratamento. pdf. Access in 06/28/2019.

BOVO JÚNIOR, Irineu. A saúde psicoemocional do pastor e as causas dos altos índices de depressão e suicídio. 2018. Dissertação de Conclusão de Curso (Mestrado em Liderança Pastoral Urbana) – UNIFIL. Londrina. 2018

CASSEMIRO, Silene L. da S. Conflitos do ministério pastoral - Um estudo de pastores em Londrina – PR. 2018. Dissertação de Conclusão de Curso (Mestrado em Liderança Pastoral Urbana) – UNIFIL. Londrina. 2018.

CASTILLO, Ana R. GL.; RECONDO, Rogéria; ASBAHR, Fernando R.; MANFRO, Gisele. Transtornos de ansiedade. Revista Brasileira de Psiquiatria. v. 22 s. 2. São Paulo. Dezembro 2000. Available at http:// www.scielo.br/ scielo.php? script= sci arttext&pid=S1516-44462000000600006. Access in 06/23/2019.

CORBAL, Betyna S. Síndrome de Burnout – Síndrome do esgotamento profissional. Previdência Social. Brasil. 2015. Available at https:// www2. camara.leg.br/ atividade-legislativa/ comissoes/ comissoes- permanentes/ cssf/ audiencias- publicas/ audiencia- publica- 2015/ audiencia-10-12-manha/ apresentacao-betyna. Access in 05/30/2019.

DEUS, Persio R.G. de. Um estudo da depressão em pastores protestantes. Ciências da Religião – História e Sociedade, São Paulo, v. 7, n. 1, 190-202, 2009. Available at http://editorarevistas.mackenzie.br/index.php/cr/article/view/1134. Access in 06/16/2019.

DUKE CLERGY HEALTH INITIATIVE. 2014 Statewide Survey of United Methodist Clergy in North Carolina. Durham. 2014. Available at https:// divinity. duke.edu/ sites/ divinity. Duke .edu/ files/ documents/ chi/ 2014%20Summary%20Report%20- 20CHI% 20Statewide%20Survey% 20of% 20United% 20Methodist% 20Clergy% 20in%20North%20Carolina%20-%20web.pdf. Access in 06/31/2019.

EVANGELICAL PRESBYTERIAN CHURCH. The Westminster Confession of Faith in Modern English. Orlando, 2010. Available at https://epc.org/wp-content/uploads/Files/1-Who-We-Are/B-About-The-EPC/WCF-ModernEnglish.pdf. Access in 01/08/2019.

FERNANDES, Márcia A.; RIBEIRO, Hellany K. P.; SANTOS. José D.M.; MONTEIRO, Claudete F.S.; COSTAL, Rosana S.; SOARES, Ricardo F.S. Prevalência dos transtornos de ansiedade como causa de afastamento de trabalhadores. Rev Bras Enferm [Internet]. 2018;71 (supl 5):2344-51. Available at http:// www.scielo.br/ pdf/ reben/ v71s5/ pt_0034-7167-reben-71-s5-2213.pdf. Access in 06/11/2019.

GAVIN, Rejane S.; REISDORFER, Emilene; GHERARDI-DONATO, Edilaine C.S.; Dos REIS, Leonardo N.; ZANETTI, Ana C.G. Associação entre depressão, estresse, ansiedade e uso de álcool entre servidores públicos. SMAD, Revista Eletrônica Saúde Mental Álcool e Drogas. (Ed. port.) v.11 n.1. Ribeirão Preto. março 2015. Available at http://pepsic.bvsalud.org/scielo.php?script=sci_arttext&pid=S1806-69762015000100002&lng=pt&nrm=iso&tlng=pt. Access in 07/19/2019.

GODOY, Rossane Frizzo de. Ansiedade, depressão e desesperança em pacientes com doença pulmonar obstrutiva crônica. Estudos & Pesquisas em Psicologia, Rio de Janeiro, v. 13, n. 3, out./dez. 2013. Available at https://www.e-publicacoes.uerj.br/index.php/revispsi/article/view/8607/6576. Access in 05/12/2020.

GOMES, Antonio M.A. Um olhar sobre depressão e religião numa perspectiva compreensiva. Estudos de Religião, São Paulo, v. 25, n. 40, 81-109, jan./jun. 2011. Available at https://www.metodista.br/revistas/revistas-ims/index.php/ER/article/viewFile/2368/2555. Access in

06/01/2019.

HOLY BIBLE, NEW INTERNATIONAL VERSION. Copyright © 1973, 1978, 1978 International Bible Society

KONKIEWITZ, Elisabete C., MAGRINELLI, Ariadne B., SALES, Dayane C. S., BENTO, Débora R. G. de M., MENEGOTTO, Elimar M. de A., LEITE, Mariana C. da C. Tópicos de Neurociência clínica. Editora UFGD. Dourados. 2010. Available at http:// files.ufgd.edu.br/ arquivos/ arquivos/ 78/ EDITORA/ T%C3% B3picos% 20de%20neuroci%C3%AAncia%20cl%C3%ADnica.pdf. Access in 06/28/2019.

LEVITAN, Michelle N.; CHAGAS, Marcos H.N.; CRIPPA, José A.S.; MANFRO, Gisele G.; HETEM, Luiz A. B.; ANDRADA, Nathalia C., SALUM, Giovanni A.; ISOLAN, Luciano; FERRARI. Maria C.F.; NARDI, Antonio E. Diretrizes da Associação Médica Brasileira para o tratamento do transtorno de ansiedade social. Revista Brasileira de Psiquiatria, v. 33, n. 3, São Paulo, setembro 2011. Available at http://www.scielo.br/pdf/rbp/v33n3/14.pdf. Access in 06/18/2019.

LOTUFO NETO, Francisco. Psiquiatria e religião: a prevalência de transtornos mentais entre ministros religiosos. 1997.Universidade de São Paulo, São Paulo, 1997. Available at http:// www.ieef.org.br/ wp-content/ uploads/ 2013/03/ PSIQUIATRIA- E-RELIGI%C3%83O-% E2% 80% 93-A-PREVAL% C3%8 ANCIA-DE- TRANSTOR- NOS -MENTAIS -ENTRE- MINISTROS-RELIGIO- SOS.pdf. Access in 06/01/2019.

LOTUFO NETO, Francisco; LOTUFO JR., Zenon; MARTINS, José C. Influências da religião sobre a saúde mental. ESETec. São Paulo. 2009. Available at https:// www.faseh.edu.br/ wp-content/ uploads/2016/02/ Influ-- ncias-da-religi--o-sobre- a-sa--de-mental-Lotufo.pdf. Access in 06/28/2019.

MELO NETO. Valfrido L. de; LÔBO, Alice P. da S.; VASCONCELOS, Juarez R. de O. Risco de suicídio e comorbidades psiquiátricas no transtorno de ansiedade generalizada. Jornal Brasileiro de Psiquiatria. v. 64 n. 4. Rio de Janeiro. Outubro/Dezembro 2015. Available at http:// www.scielo.br/ scielo.php?script= sci_arttext&pid=S0047-20852015000400259. Access in 06/26/2019.

MINISTÉRIO DA SAÚDE DO BRASIL ORGANIZAÇÃO PAN-AMERICANA DA SAÚDE NO BRASIL. Doenças relacionadas ao Trabalho – Manual de Procedimentos para os Serviços de Saúde. Ministério da Saúde. Brasília/DF. 2001. Available at http:// bvsms.saude.gov.br/ bvs/ publicacoes/ doencas relacionadas trabalho manual procedimentos.pdf. Access in 07/31/2019.

MORENO, Fernanda N., GIL, Gislaine P., HADDAD, Maria do Carmo L., VANNUCHI, Marli T.O. Estratégias e intervenções no enfrentamento da síndrome de burnout. Revista de Enfermagem da UERJ. v. 19 s. 1. Rio de Janeiro. Janeiro/Março 2011. Available at http://www.facenf.uerj.br/v19n1/v19n1a23.pdf. Access in 06/30/2019.

PIOTROWSKI, C. The status of the Beck Anxiety Inventory in contemporary research. *Psychol Rep.* 85 (1): 261–2. 1999. Available at https://www.ncbi.nlm.nih.gov/pubmed/10575991. Access in 05/12/2020

PORTAL DA EDUCAÇÃO TECNOLOGIA EDUCACIONAL LTDA. A Síndrome De Burnout: Aspectos Relevantes Para O Mundo Do Trabalho. São Paulo. Available at https://www.portaleducacao.com.br/conteudo/artigos/psicologia/a-sindrome-de-burnout- aspectos- relevantes- para- o- mundo- do- trabalho/27982. Access in 08/01/2019.

PORTAL DO GOVERNO BRASILEIRO – MINISTÉRIO DA SAÚDE. Depressão: causas, sintomas, tratamentos, diagnóstico e prevenção. Available at http://www.saude.gov.br/saude-de-a-z/saude-mental/depressao. Access in 06/18/2019.

PORTAL DO GOVERNO BRASILEIRO – MINISTÉRIO DA SAÚDE. Síndrome de Burnout: causas, sintomas, tratamentos, diagnóstico e prevenção. Available at http://www.saude.gov.br/ saude-de-a-z/ saude-mental/ sindrome-de-burnout. Access in 06/13/2019.

RIBEIRO, Hellany K. P.; SANTOS, José D. M.; MONTEIRO, Claudete F. de S.; COSTA, Rosana dos S.; SOARES, Ricardo F.S. Prevalência dos transtornos de ansiedade como causa de afastamento de trabalhadores. Revista Brasileira de Enfermagem. v. 71 s. 5. Brasília. 2018. Available at http:// www. scielo.br/ scielo. php? script= sci_arttext& pid= S0034-71672018001102213&lng= en&nrm= iso& tlng= pt. Access in 06/23/2019.

SANTOS, Ana Cristina de O.; HONÓRIO, Luiz C. As Dimensões da Síndrome de Burnout no Trabalho dos Pastores da Igreja Presbiteriana do Brasil em Minas Gerais. XXXVIII Encontro da Associação Nacional de Pós-Graduação e Pesquisa em Administração – ANPAD. Rio de Janeiro, 2014. Available at http:// www. anpad.org.br/admin/pdf/2014_EnANPAD_GPR359.pdf. Access in 04/23/2019.

SOEIRO, Rachel E.; COLOMBO, Elisabetta S.; FERREIRA, Marianne H.F.; GUIMARÃES, Paula S.A.; BOTEGA, Neury J.; DALGALARRONDO, Paulo. Religião e transtornos mentais em pacientes internados em um hospital geral universitário. Caderno de Saúde Pública. v. 24 n. 4. Rio de Janeiro. Abril 2008. Available at http:// www.scielo.br/scielo.php?script=sci_arttext&pid=S0102-311X 2008000400009&lang=en. Access in 06/22/2019.

SOUZA, Fabio G.M. Tratamento da depressão. Revista Brasileira de Psiquiatria, vol. 21, s. 1, São Paulo, Maio 1999. Available at http:// www.scielo.br/ scielo. php?script= sci_arttext& pid= S1516-44461999000500005. Access in 07/18/2019.

TRIGO, Telma R., TENG, Chei T., HALLAK, Jaime E.C. Síndrome de burnout ou estafa profissional e os transtornos psiquiátricos. Revista de Psiquiatria Clínica. v. 34 n. 5, Brasil, 2007. Available at http:// www. scielo.br/ pdf/ rpc/ v34n5/ a04v34n5.pdf. Access in 06/30/2019.

VALLADA FILHO, Homero P., LAFER, Beny. Genética

e fisiopatologia dos transtornos depressivos. Revista Brasileira de Psiquiatria. v. 21 s. 1. São Paulo. Maio 1999. Available at http:// www.scielo.br/ scielo.php? script= sci_arttext& pid=S1516-44461999000500004. Access in 06/29/2019.

VARGAS, Elvira L. Um olhar para a família pastoral. 2018. Dissertação de Conclusão de Curso (Mestrado em Liderança Pastoral Urbana) – UNIFIL. Londrina. 2018.

VASCONCELOS, Juarez R. de O.; LÔBO, Alice P. da S.; MELO NETO, Valfrido L. Risco de suicídio e comorbidades psiquiátricas no transtorno de ansiedade generalizada. Jornal Brasileiro de Psiquiatria. v. 64 n. 4. Rio de Janeiro. Out/Dez. 2015. Available at http://www.scielo.br/scielo.php?script=sci_arttext&pid=S0047-20852015000400259. Access in 06/28/2019.

VOLLET, Angela B. D. L.; WIGGERS, Eliz M.. A relação entre espiritualidade, saúde e pasicologia: uma pesquisa bibliográfica. Itajai. 2019. Personal comunication received by drdelcio@hotmail.com in 07/12/2017.

WORLD HEALTH ORGANIZATION - WHO. Depression

and other common mental disorders: global health estimates. Geneva. 2017. Available at http:// apps. who. int/ iris/ bitstream/ 10665/254610/1/ WHO-MSD-MER-2017.2-eng.pdf. Access in 06/28/2019.

WORLD HEALTH ORGANIZATION. Burn-out um "fenômeno ocupacional": Classificação Internacional de Doenças. Genebra, 2019. Available at https:// www.who.int/mental_health/evidence/burn-out/en/. Access in 08/01/2019.

WORLD HEALTH ORGANIZATION. Preventing suicide – A global imperative. Genebra, 2014. Available at https:// www.who.int/ mental health/ suicide-prevention/world report 2014/en/. Access in 08/01/2019.

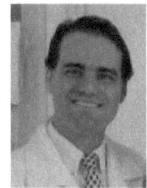

Delcio Torres Amorim Junior. Brazilian Presbyterian pastor and physician graduated in Medicine from the Londrina State University (Brazil), medical residency in General Surgery at São Paulo Pontifical Catholic University, Master in Business Administration at Fundação Getúlio Vargas. Theology from the Hosanna Theological Seminary and a Master's in Theology from the Philadelphia University Center – UniFil. Professor in the postgraduate course in psychoanalysis and member of the academic and scientific board at the International Institute of Psychoanalysis. Creator and coordinator of "The Potter's House", a comprehensive health care program for pastors, priests, Christian religious ministers and their families. Currently praticing medicine and pastoral ministry in Brazil.

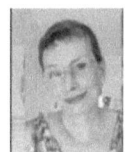
"Despite being a psychiatrist for 40 years, I was surprised by the content presented by Dr. Delcio Torres Amorim Jr in this study. Religious ministers' lives is shrouded in a mist of mystery for us lay people. The mystery feeds the most diverse fantasies. Such fantasies are addressed with clarity, faith, and science in this book. The clear and lucid approach presented is certainly very useful for mental health professionals, when involved in caring for this pressured and suffering population of pastors, their families and religious in general. The examples taken from the biblical accounts are very interesting and evaluated in the light of modern psychiatry and psychology. I loved Reading it!!!!". Dr. Angela Bertoni de Miranda, psychiatrist in São Paulo (Brazil).

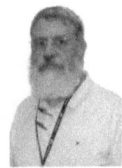
"This text deserves careful reading, study and reflection by religion ministers, seminarians, health professionals and leaders of religious communities. The main mental disorders are described from a medical, psychological and biblical perspective. It points to the behavioral, psychological and spiritual care that can favor health and protect it. I congratulate Dr. Delcio for such careful work that he will undoubtedly contribute to the pastoral ministry in Brazil. Prof. Dr. Francisco Lotufo Neto, psychologist and psychiatrist, associate professor at the School of Medicine and the Institute of Psychology at the University of São Paulo (Brazil)

www.ingramcontent.com/pod-product-compliance
Lightning Source LLC
Chambersburg PA
CBHW031446210526
45464CB00005B/2350